BANG!

masturbation for people of all genders and abilities

vic liu

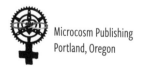

Microcosm Publishing
Portland, Oregon

Bang! Masturbation for People of All Genders and Abilities
© Vic Liu 2021
This edition © Microcosm Publishing, 2021
Contributions remain the property of their individual creators
This is Microcosm #564
ISBN #9781621063858
First Edition, June 8, 2021
Cover and Design by Vic Liu

Microcosm Publishing
2752 N Williams Ave
Portland, OR 97227
(503)799-2698
Other zines, books, stickers, patches, pins, posters, t-shirts, DVDs, & more:
www.Microcosm.Pub

To join the ranks of high-class stores that feature Microcosm titles, talk to your rep: In the U.S. Como (Atlantic), Fujii (Midwest), Book Travelers West (Pacific), Turnaround in Europe, Manda/UTP in Canada, New South in Australia/New Zealand, and GPS in Asia, India, Africa, and South America. We are sold in the gift market by Gifts of Nature and by Faire.

Did you know that you can buy our books directly from us at sliding scale rates? Support a small, independent publisher and pay less than Amazon's price at www.Microcosm.Pub

Global labor conditions are bad, and our roots in industrial Cleveland in the 70s and 80s made us appreciate the need to treat workers right. Therefore, our books are MADE IN THE USA.

Library of Congress Cataloging-in-Publication Data

Names: Liu, Vic, author.
Title: Bang! : masturbation for people of all genders / Vic Liu.
Description: Portland : Microcosm Publishing, 2021. | Includes bibliographical references. | Summary: "Want to know how to masturbate? Here's your guide. Whether you're jerking the gherkin, flicking the bean, or something in between, masturbation doesn't have to be a taboo topic. This straightforward, unapologetic illustrated guide to self-pleasure will teach you what you need to know to get to know your own body. This inclusive manual covers basic anatomy, techniques, mindsets, orgasms, troubleshooting, and a wide range of the tools and toys. There are sections on debunking myths, exploring your body for the first time, sex toys, tips from trans people for trans people, and a section on masturbating when you have a physical disability and a caretaker that's written by disabled folks. You'll also learn about the history of anti-masturbation stigma, some thought-provoking data, and how to teach your kids healthy attitudes toward masturbation. Perfect for the pent-up teens and adults of all ages alike! Overcome physical and emotional obstacles to discover the stress-relieving potential and joy of unpartnered sex. Includes writing and illustrations by Vic Liu, Nina Chausow, Alex Tait, Clare Edgeman, Leah Holmes, Sam Dusing, Patrick Wiedeman, Rebecca Bedell, Lafayette Matthews, Andrew Gurza, and Angus Andrews"-- Provided by publisher.
Identifiers: LCCN 2020050996 | ISBN 9781621063858 (paperback)
Subjects: LCSH: Masturbation. | Mind and body.
Classification: LCC HQ447 .L58 2021 | DDC 306.77/2--dc23
LC record available at https://lccn.loc.gov/2020050996

HOW TO USE THIS BOOK

1 Remember that you're the commander-in-chief of your body. You run the show. You make the call.

2 Read it in whatever order or way you like. Take what you find helpful or valuable. Leave the rest.

Our Terminology

For trans and intersex people, genitalia can be a huge source of dysphoria. Much of this book was written by cis people, often defaulting to scientific terms like penis and clitoris. Feel free to cross out any terms and write in your own! We've strived together for inclusive language, but please know that whatever your body looks like, however you feel or talk about it, you can own it and enjoy it. You deserve every bit of radical self-love.

CONTENTS

setting
the mood

an introduction

DEAREST READER,

Take a moment to appreciate your body.

Thank your genitals. Your vagina, your clitoris, your penis, or your testicles. Definitely your anus. They are all working naturally, simply, and exactly as they should. Nothing is wrong with them, whatever they look like, feel like, or allow you to experience.

You may be smiling to yourself, thinking about the orgasm you had this morning. You may be cringing, because it's difficult to say any of these words even in your head.

For people on every part of this and any spectrum: this book is for you.

Masturbation is a time and space you give yourself to be present with and inside your body. You deserve and are allowed to feel the highest level of physical pleasure, whatever that means to you at this moment. Inside of that space, there is no room for judgment or expectations, whether imposed from the outside or hiding deep in the corners of your mind.

Masturbation is not a competition or a destination.

It is a practice, and it will only improve as you give yourself permission to take the time that you need, create a space that makes you truly comfortable, and explore tools to help grow your experience.

Orgasms are great, but they are no more important than crafting a masturbation practice that listens to the needs, responses, and questions of your body as you examine what pleasure and sensation feel like in the moment.

When you're ready, let's get started.

myths about masturbation

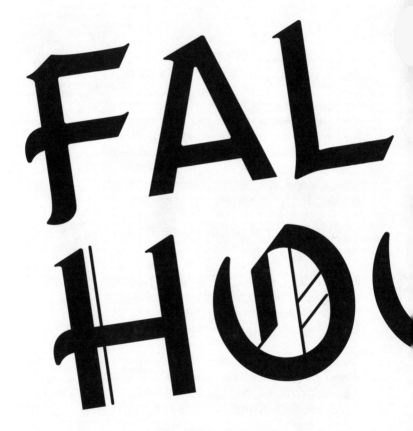

FAL
HOO

Society can get very inventive when it comes up with reasons for people not to touch themselves.

Masturbation myths of the olden days say that your palms will grow hairy, you'll go blind, and that you're killing little mini babies every time you ejaculate outside of a vagina. While these myths may sound ridiculous now, many of today's falsehoods debunked here are just as far from the truth.

Masturbation does not take your virginity.

Virginity is a powerful social construct that has a tendency to spread. Virginity was invented to ensure marriage was a clean financial contract with clear inheritance lines; in other words, to make sure people only had babies with the people they married so that money stayed in the core family. But the idea it uses to control people, that sex is dirty or sinful, spreads beyond contact between penis and vagina, into areas like, *if I touch myself, am I sullied?*

Try to be mindful of and deliberate about the beliefs that can lurk on the fringes of your mind. Why does virginity matter to you? Do you connect sexuality with moral impurity? Do you have a religious perspective?

We, and medical professionals, can assure you that masturbation is perfectly natural, normal, and healthy. What we can't do is change your inner narrative about what masturbation means to you. That is entirely up to you. But pages 72–79 might be helpful.

Childhood masturbation is normal.

Childhood masturbation is absolutely normal, beginning on average between the ages of 2 and 6. During these years, children often use masturbation to explore their body. Normal can range from not at all to several times a day.

Consider consulting a pediatrician in cases where masturbation interferes with the child's ability to live a normal life, if the child is using objects to masturbate that might be harmful, or if you have any questions in general. For more info, take a look at pages 92–97.

Masturbation doesn't cause infertility or erectile dysfunction.

Many scientific studies have found no connection between masturbation and infertility.

Because sperm is produced every day, people who have testicles don't have to worry about masturbation reducing their sperm count.

IMAGE: A man lies dying from masturbation.
The Secret Companion, R J Brodie, London, 1845.

Overwhelming amounts of scientific data have also concluded that masturbation does not result in erectile dysfunction.

That is, there is absolutely no correlation between infertility, erectile dysfunction, and masturbation. Nada. Zip. Zero.

Masturbation during menstruation is healthy.

It is absolutely safe and healthy to masturbate during your period. We would recommend removing a tampon if you have one in before any penetration. If you are concerned about mess, consider laying down a towel for worry-free easy cleaning after the fact.

Masturbation is not a red flag in a relationship.

Masturbation within a relationship does not mean that the relationship is not sexually fulfilling. For some, masturbation does not replace partnered sex, but instead is a completely separate sexual practice. Just because you ate breakfast, doesn't mean you can't have lunch.

Masturbation can also be a valuable supplement to partnered sex. It allows people to figure out their sexual bodies as individuals, before adding a whole

IMAGE: 18th Century, an unhappy wife complains to an official about her husband's impotence, using a dildo as evidence. *Hamse-i Atai*

Now that

other body and brain to the mix. Masturbation can also help with unequal sexual appetites within a relationship. Sometimes when I go out to a fancy meal and the plates are small, I'll get a bite to eat later. The fancy meal with the smaller plate was still absolutely wonderful, and that bite to eat later allows me to have the best of both worlds. Masturbation can also help if situationally it's hard for the two people to have sex as much as one (or both) of them would like.

For what it's worth, a 2009 study found that the masturbation frequency of women (most likely referring to cis women of all sexual orientations) is not statistically affected by whether or not they are in a relationship, single, or married.[1]

that we've gotten
all straightened out...

what masturbation can do for you

THE PERKS
OF PLAYING

Besides the obvious effect of making you less of a horny toad, masturbation can...

1 Strengthen tone in pelvic and anal areas, including the pelvic floor.

2 Improve sexual stamina if you practice delaying orgasm.

3 Relieve muscle tension and menstrual cramps by relaxing the pelvic muscles.

Help you sleep by releasing serotonin and endorphins.

Improve circulation to your pelvic area.

Reduce stress, tension from headaches, and neck pain.

Improve self-esteem and body image. Masturbation helps you discover all the wonderful things your genitals can do.

Help out your sexual relations. Let's put it this way: If you learn how your body works, you can tell your partner exactly what they're doing right and what they haven't figured out yet.

All without the risk of STIs or pregnancy!

getting in the right mental zone

HEADSPACE

Surrender to the Spank Bank

Before getting physical, many people struggle to get past the mental roadblock. One of our authors suggests collecting the mental imagery that turns you on into a 'personal porno' to help put you in the mood and declutter your mind.

Everyone is turned on by things they don't understand, things that might surprise you or feel embarrassing. No one should judge their own tendencies. We assure you we all fantasize about some weird stuff. Starting with the hang-up that many people have about masturbation itself, and working to cultivate a positive and open headspace for sex and pleasure is incredibly important.

That being said, you need to be safe and keep others safe in this pursuit, so if you have thoughts or fantasies regarding people who do not consent or cannot give consent (for example, due to age or incapacitation) we encourage you to reach out to a mental health professional.

Be the O, don't seek the O

It can be frustrating when you feel like you can't achieve orgasm. First-timers and people having trouble finding their route to orgasm, be patient! The less time spent working towards a "goal," the better. While ending a masturbation with an orgasm seems like a convenient closing point, the rush to the finish can also remove all of the valuable and enjoyable time in which to explore and learn about what pleasure feels, looks, and smells like in each body.

Masturbation should be more of a space of exploration than a journey to the end. While sometimes you need to just rub one out, masturbation can and should be a judgment-free zone for everyone to learn what turns them on. Different things work better for different people. For example, some people use lube every time they masturbate. Others, for example, people with circumcised penises, may enjoy the friction caused by a different type of stimulation. For some people, masturbation comes very easily both physically and mentally, and for others, adding sensations such as porn or toys into the mix can be really helpful for sinking into the right space.

Consume as much research as you can, and look for scientifically backed and factual resources that come from unbiased sources. Have fun, be informed, be strong, and pursue pleasure!

getting down to business

a geographical menu

TWID
BITS

ODLY

In the next few pages, you'll find what we like to call a menu. See what appeals to you, and leave the rest.

Feel free to scribble and draw all over these pages, to make the diagrams reflect you. A little fact that porn and many people aren't aware of: genitalia spans a huge spectrum of size and shape. Do you have more folds there than what you see in porn? Cool. More skin? Awesome. Is your clit bigger? Your testicles lower? Maybe you're intersex or have had gender affirmation surgeries, and you have a combination of different parts of the last four pages. In all cases, you and your genitals are pretty great.

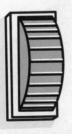

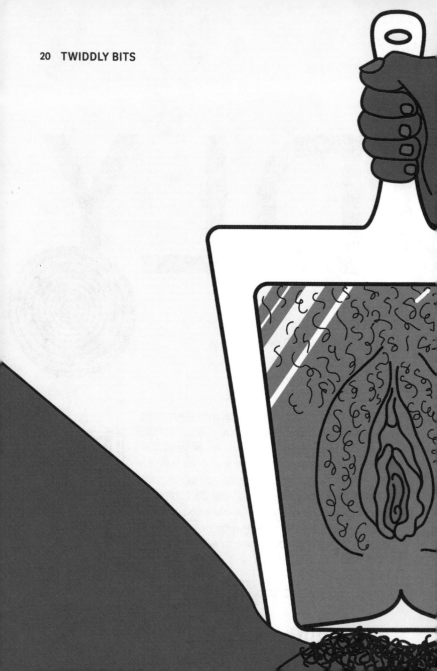

Mons

The fatty tissue on top of your pubic bone might not be the most sensitive of the bits, but that doesn't mean you should ignore it. Vibration and even just pressure can be super nice when applied to the mons, particularly while stimulating other erogenous zones.

Labia

The labia can be a great place to start when going solo. Explore your labia with your fingers: rubbing, pulling, even twisting. Using your hands to explore, or even getting a vibrator (vibe) involved while playing with your labia, can be a great warm-up to your clit, or just a pleasurable adventure for its own sake.

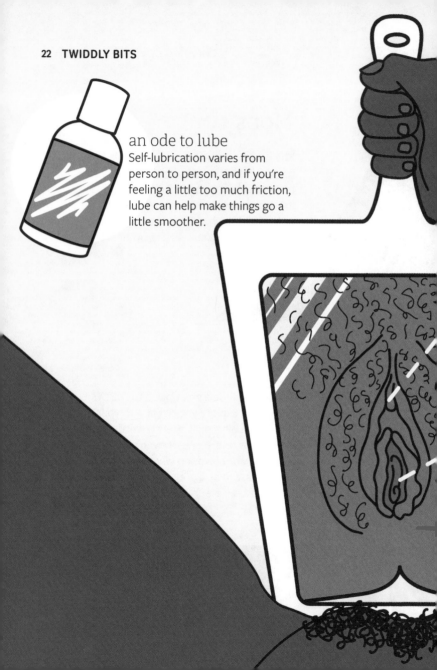

an ode to lube
Self-lubrication varies from person to person, and if you're feeling a little too much friction, lube can help make things go a little smoother.

Clitoris

Sometimes it's best to approach the clit from the side, back, or front. Point is, you don't always need to directly stimulate your clit to stimulate your clit. In fact, sometimes direct stimulation can be a bit much. Use your fingers (or a vibe) and build up to the level of stimulation that gets you going.

Vagina

First off, don't get too preoccupied with the G-Spot (or more accurately, area); instead just do what feels good. For some people that might be the G-area, a cluster of nerves located on the front wall, towards your belly. For others, general penetration might be preferable. Exploring the inside with your fingers, a vibrator, or a dildo is great whether you're seeking arousal or just information about your body. Not everyone likes penetration, and that is completely okay and normal!

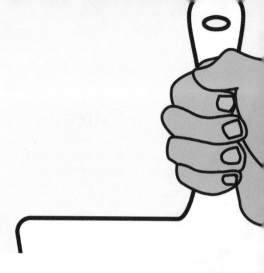

Glans (Head)

Most of the nerve endings in a penis are found in the head, aka glans. Lube can be your best friend here, although pre-cum can also serve as lubrication for this section of your genitalia. You can utilize your thumb with strokes down the head, circles around the tip of the glans, and any combination of the two. Stroking off and onto the head, you also stimulate the corona or head of your penis. Regardless of whether or not you have a foreskin, this spot is super sensitive and worth some exploration with various pressures, speeds, and lubrication levels.

Frenulum

This is the largest concentration of nerves on your penis. Try something as simple as light tickles while stimulating other parts of your genitalia, or alternating between more vigorous approaches. Firm pressure, stroking, tickling… experiment with ranges of stimulation and how you can use the sensitivity of this particular part to switch things up.

Shaft

Friction is your friend here. Not too much, of course. But a vigorous stroke that emphasizes the pressure between your hand and your shaft can be a great place to start. Experiment with pacing and styles of strokes. Try long twisting strokes, combined with a hand held tightly around the base of your shaft, or cupping of your testicles. The combinations are endless!

uncircumcised?
You're probably more
sensitive, you lucky dog.

Testicles

The scrotum has lots of nerves, and your
testicles can be super sensitive. So don't
ignore them when it comes to getting funky
with yourself. Cupping, gentle pulling, and
general fondling can be a great place to start
to bring your balls into your self-love routine.

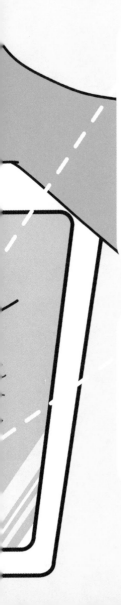

Inguinal Canals

Penetration of these canals is called muffing, common among trans women but potentially explosive for any penis owner. And yes, it's safe! Start slow and careful; finger around the base of the penis for the openings, then push the skin inward/upward. Massaging the concentrated nerve endings inside the canals can give a spark to your playtime, though pleasure varies widely from person to person.

Perineum

This magical area between the penis and anus is incredibly sensitive to pressure and massage. Rubbing this area provides external stimulation of the prostate, and is a great way to start exploring your prostate if you aren't ready for internal exploration.

Nip it

Nipples can be hotbeds of nerve endings, but it really depends on how you're wired. Play around with everything from tickling, flicking, twisting, and even slapping. It depends on how sensitive your nipples are; some nipple owners even like incorporating pain or more sharp sensations for ultimate stimulation. You can really get creative here.

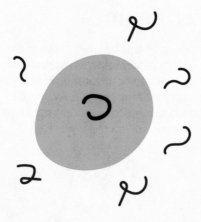

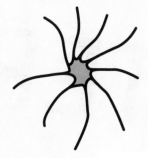

In the Bud

Everyone's got an anus! There are many nerve endings to be found both around the outside and just inside the anus. Start off slow and with smaller toys, and relaaaxxxx your muscles down there. Explore various pressures, and if you're ready to go in, make sure to lube up. If you're lucky enough to have a prostate, it's a super-center of nerve endings that can be stimulated both through massage of the perineum and through internal stimulation with either a finger or a toy. And again, lube, lube, lube!

A few safety rules: anything that goes in should have a flared base (there are plenty of rectum x-rays on the internet that agree). Also, beware of numbing creams. Listen to what your body tells you, including pain.

let's launch you off

MASTER

One of the most exciting and terrifying things about masturbating is that there is no secret formula.

IMAGE: Saturn Apollo Program

DEBATE

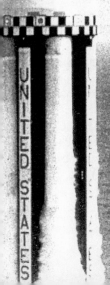

There is no password that can be passed surreptitiously from one person to the next that magically unlocks their orgasm potential.

Anything learned about masturbation from the outside really only serves as a jumping-off point for understanding the unique desires and quirks of each body. That being said, hearing about other people's experiences, challenges, and successes can be empowering and enlightening.

Penile Pleasure

Make yourself erect by moving the head of your penis around in circles or rubbing it against your leg. Grip your shaft so that your index finger falls on your frenulum (see page 23) and your thumb falls opposite. Tighten your thumb and index finger while moving them around each other in a circular motion. When you are erect, move your hand up and down your shaft. Lubrication is completely optional—if it's dry, the friction between your thumb and head, palm and shaft will feel good. If you are using lube or lotion, the feeling will be more diffuse and good in a different way. Water is abrasive. If you are in the shower, use soap to keep your hands lubricated.

If you want to minimize clean-up, maybe plan out where you are going to ejaculate before you start, rather than in the moment. Your landing pad could be a tissue, toilet paper (which is flushable), the shower, or even a condom.

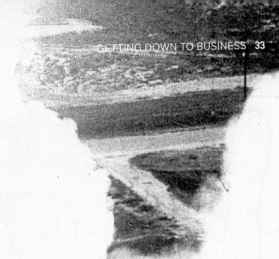

Cliteracy

Start by lying in a comfortable position. Lying on the back or side allows easy access to the clitoris, while lying on the belly offers the opportunity to introduce an external object such as a pillow for further stimulation. Spread the labia, and use two fingers to start to circle the clitoris. Maybe add some lube if you'd like! The head of the clitoris can be very sensitive, so rubbing circles around it and moving the clitoral hood up and down, or even rubbing the clitoris through fabric, can provide less intense stimulation. Start slowly, and get progressively faster and add more pressure if that feels good.

cum first, clean later

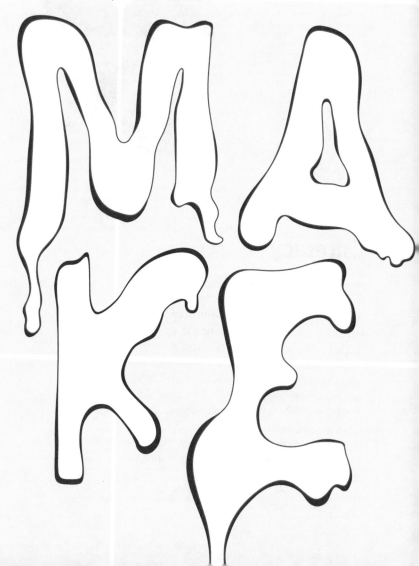

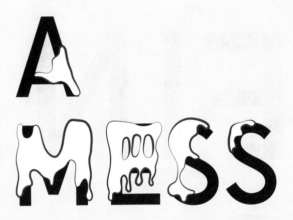

A MESS

There very well may be something to clean up when all is said and done. Everyone differs when it comes to how to react, but it's definitely good to approach wiping yourself up with something soft and without shame.

Masturbating in the bath or shower might set the mood and help take clean-up off your mind, allowing you to let go and focus on the moment.

Afterwards, especially if you have a shorter urethra, it's a good idea to pee to decrease your risk of getting a UTI. There is no need to use soap to clean up, but if you want to, use plain, unperfumed soap so that you don't mess with the healthy balance of bacteria around your genitals.

masturbating while trans

FIND

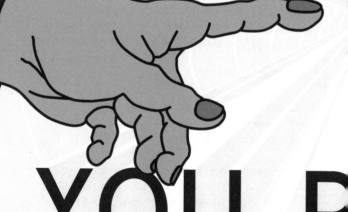

YOU-P

Inside illustrations by Lafayette Matthews

DING

Rebecca Bedell and Lafayette Matthews

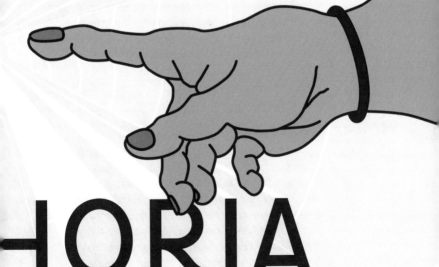

HORIA

Being your own body
Transmasculine

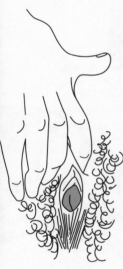

For me, as a transgender man, masturbation is all about affirmation and discovering new ways to love my body.

If you start testosterone, one of the first changes you will notice is clitoral enlargement (between one and five centimeters) with increased sensitivity and sex drive. You may enjoy masturbating the same way you always have, or you may find that pulling gives you more sensation. It's *your* clit/junk/peen/dick, so play around with it and find what feels good! Don't be afraid to use your extra hole, but make sure to get well-lubricated because testosterone can cause vaginal dryness. You can also try "pack and play" devices or masturbation sleeves, like the Shotpocket Sleeve.

There are a few possible bottom surgeries for transmasculine folks, including metoidioplasty (meta) and phalloplasty (phallo), which can also include testicular implants. Meta releases your junk from the clitoral hood to create a small penis, while phalloplasty constructs a penis using a donor graft from your arm or leg. Your post-op sensation may vary on the technique and recovery time as the nerves regenerate, but masturbation can become more pleasurable and affirming.

Transfeminine

In my experience as a trans woman, pleasure can be simple AND complicated. Masturbation is an adventure. But it can all be awesome.

For transfeminine folks, your genitals might experience any range of changes, depending on whether/when you start estrogen and/or testosterone blockers. Some trans femmes, not all, have trouble staying hard after hormones; if this happens to you, fear not! With estrogen, your nipples may become more sensitive, and you might even find yourself able to have multiple orgasms. You might love the penetrative feeling of muffing (see page 25), though if you tuck your testicles into the inguinal canals, they can get desensitized. You can always explore your prostate. If your penis/girlcock/clit/bio-strap-on does stay soft, it'll still feel great to massage the head.

For most post-vaginoplasty and/or labiaplasty trans femmes, sexual results vary widely. Your new vagina will likely be raw and sensitive at first, as you're regularly dilating, and your clitoris may be anywhere from so sensitive it's almost painful, to very insensitive. You probably will not self-lubricate, so have lube handy, but you might still ejaculate liquid. Be careful, take it slow, and see what feels good. Have at it, you sexy femme!

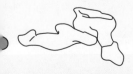

Let's face it, being trans can make pleasure a much touchier subject.

Or less touch-y, if your dysphoria makes it hard to touch and enjoy your genitals. Maybe the feeling of "this isn't what my body should be" creeps over you when you start, or crashes in after you come. You're not alone, nor are you forever stuck in a void between who you are and how your genitals are gendered. If you decide surgery is for you, we support you 100%. But this section focuses on ways to enjoy your body as it is, simply because it's your body. Consider these tips from the field: a handful of reminders to ground yourself as you edge closer to euphoria.

Re-Approach, Re-Discover

If you're comfortable, run your hands over every inch of your skin. Flip back to "Dear Reader" and "Tingly Bits." It's always worth doing: say hello and thank you to your body and all its curves, hairs, soft parts, wet parts, sensitive parts. Allow these fleshy discoveries to get you amped up.

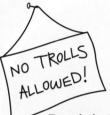

NO TROLLS ALLOWED!

Banish the Comments Section

First, you don't need every cis-het porn trope or transphobic joke replaying in your mind when you're rubbing one out. No one invited them. Try to shut out the voices and be in the moment. Lock the door and shut the blinds; any tricks that will help you feel unwatched. Pretend there are no other humans—you're the first—and you're so fucking excited to explore your marvelous body and what it can do!

What Feels Good Is Good

When your fingers or toy hits a nerve in the right way, gets a sweet shiver going, let yourself smile. Feel it. Does it feel good? Let it be good. Let pleasure itself be the sex appeal that keeps you rubbing and stroking because it's just so wonderful that your nerves feel this, that your own touch can flood you with endorphins. You deserve every bit of goodness. Your body has so much to offer you.

Flip the Thinking

You know how society has attached labels to certain kinds of bodies. You've seen what society thinks "women's bodies" (for instance) look like, and maybe you see yourself and go "this isn't what a woman's body looks like, so I'm not a woman." But that's putting outside opinions before your own truth—it's backwards. Shut out those voices, and start with what you know is true: "I'm a woman, so this is what a woman's body looks like." If it helps, look in the mirror and compliment yourself. Say, "this is a woman's body" (if you're a woman) or "this is a man's body" (if you're a man). Say "this is my body and it's beautiful" (no matter your gender). Hearing yourself say it will help you believe it.

Fantasize With Love

Fantasizing that your body looks different or has different parts can be a huge turn-on—but if you do that every time, you risk getting hit by dysphoria when you come back to reality. But keeping one foot (or finger) in reality doesn't have to kill the mood. Like many people whose bodies don't match what we're told they're "supposed" to be—cuties with disabilities, we see you—let us trans folks try this: love your body for what it can do, rather than focusing on what it can't.

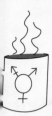

Creature Comforts

Know your triggers and your comforts. You might tend to avoid certain types of porn, positions, or sensations. If you tend to get waves of post-come sads, fluff up your self-aftercare routine. Maybe you need to burrito in a blanket after you come, or maybe you whip on some boxers or hop straight into the shower. Maybe you've been riding a kinky fantasy until you scream, but what you need after is fuzzy slippers and tea—that's okay! Learn, and treat yourself right.

New Ways to Touch

Mindfulness is all well and good, but at the end of the day it's about where you touch your body and how. Don't assume the same routine you used before transition will still feel the best—in fact, get ready to discover new, trans-tastic ways to fuck yourself! Feel around for new ways to touch; try new toys and vibrators. Remember: all shapes, sizes, softness and hardness of genitalia are sexy. Above all else, rocking what you've got is sexy.

Bon voyage, explorer!

**tips for touching with
a physical disability**

Andrew Gurza and Angus Andrews

SETTING UP FOR SOLO SEX

Inside illustrations by Angus Andrews

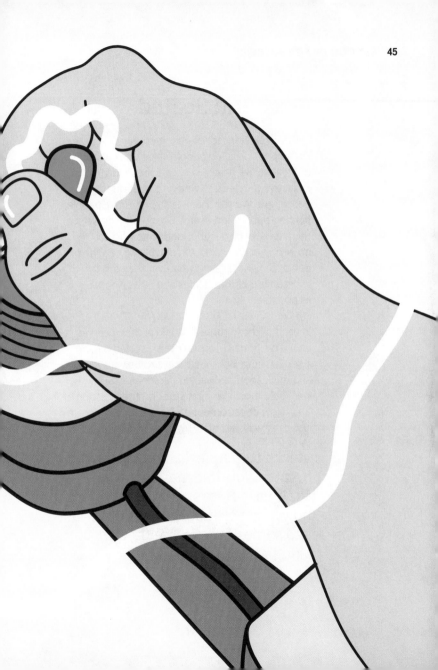

Sexy and Seated

Let's be real honest about something. When we think about disabled people, if we think about them at all, we have a very specific vision in our collective minds as to who and what disabled people are: We see them as strong, brave people fighting oppression in an ableist world, or we see them as sweet, cherubic innocents who can do no wrong in the world. Or, maybe, we see them as heroic figures doing whatever they can to overcome their disabilities and be as normal as possible.

In each of those three disabled archetypes, we would never dare consider the disabled person a sexual being. But... if we were to take a second and think about a disabled person masturbating, we would most likely get stuck on the question of how. How does someone who uses a wheelchair and can't walk get off? How does that work?

Maybe this all feels familiar to you because you, like me, are a wheelchair user. Here's a step-by-step on how a wheelchair user might get off, and some of the issues that might go along with that.

PLEASE DO NOT DISTURB

Find Some Alone Time

Sometimes, being disabled and being a wheelchair user means that you have attendant care workers with you all the time, or constantly coming in and out of your space, and this can make any privacy, let alone sexy private time, difficult to obtain. Look for a moment when you are totally alone, if you can (this may not be possible because you may need help to prepare to masturbate). When your attendant has left or at nighttime are often good times to explore self-pleasure as a disabled person. Whenever it is, find some time that is not rushed due to your care needs, and if you have to schedule it in, so that your attendants know that on this day and time you'll need help masturbating, that's okay, too.

Ask Your Personal Caregiver to Help You Set Up

As a wheelchair user, I am unable to do certain self-pleasure and masturbation things on my own. When we think about someone masturbating, we probably assume that they can take their pants off on their own, right? Well, I can't take my pants off and I need help to do that, so I may have to ask my attendant or caregiver for assistance in setting me up to self-pleasure. This can sometimes be super embarrassing or uncomfortable, but remember that they are there to help you set up, and to make the experience as accessible as possible for you. Don't be afraid to tell your attendant: "I want to masturbate by myself. Can you help me set up in my space so I can do that?"

Don't Worry About Technique

A lot of wheelchair users, such as those with cerebral palsy or muscular dystrophy, or those who acquired disability via an injury, have very limited dexterity in their hands and forearms. This may make it difficult for them to assume masturbatory positions with their hands in order to stroke their penis or finger their clitoris.

When I first learned to masturbate, I didn't do it the traditional way that most penis-havers do it. I used my thumb and forefinger to create friction as I was unable (and am still unable) to pump my penis. Whatever way that you do it, whether you come or not, is totally okay! Try not to get too far in your own head about it, about how it is supposed to look, and just try to enjoy the moment. If it doesn't look like what you've seen in popular pornography, that is perfectly fine.

Tilt Back and Take a Load Off

As a power wheelchair user, you might have a chair with the ability to tilt back. This can be a great advantage to masturbation (if you choose to do so in your chair) because you can stretch out some and have easier access to your genitalia so that you can explore yourself with ease. Most non-disabled people don't jerk off at a 90 degree angle, and neither should you. If tilting isn't available or masturbating in your chair isn't an option, you might want to ask your caregiver to put you in bed.

Capitalization Nation

As a queer, incomplete paraplegic, horny cartoonist, I often have to give myself some ~alone time~ to reset and reconnect with myself. So here are my three go-to tips for having sex with chronic pain, fatigue, and limited sensation.

Expanding Your Erotic Imagination

A major piece of the disability and sex puzzle for me revolves around physical sensation (and more specifically, my lack of). I lack a lot of sensation in my body. I have no feeling at all in my feet or legs below the knees, minimal feeling in my thighs and upper legs, and dulled sensation in my hip and groin area. This is to say that while I can feel touch in erogenous places, I often need very specific types of touch to really feel it.

This is where brain waves really kick in. Sometimes, to feel sexy, you've got to think sexy. Getting yourself into a headspace where you can feel turned on just by knowing what you're doing to yourself is a major part of getting off (especially when you're going solo!). Our minds are a powerful thing. Do a little sexy homework: Look into what really turns you on, and go there in your mind.

Explore any part of your body that feels good! And remember that sex and masturbation can be defined any way you want.

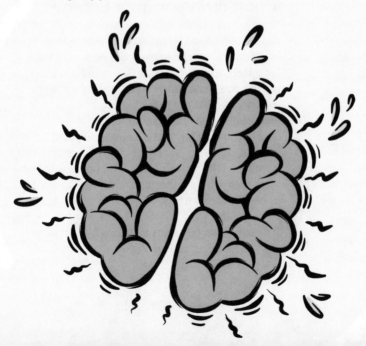

Capitalizing on Your Energy

I'm exhausted and sore pretty much 24/7. My 10-minute commute to and from work feels like an athletic event; my showers, a chore; I'm tired writing this sentence. It can be physically and emotionally draining to live with chronic pain and fatigue, and figuring out how to make time and find energy for masturbating is perhaps my biggest barrier to getting off. It's a real drag sometimes. If this feels close to home for you, dear reader, here is the good news: you can do this—you deserve this.

The big workaround isn't in making more time or energy, it's about capitalizing on what you've got.

If you do best in the morning after a big sleep,
I can assure you it's an amazing way to start your
day. If you find yourself needing a nap before or
after, carving out an extra few minutes for some
(get) down time with yourself may be all you really
need. Capitalize on your good days or your good
moments on otherwise medium days. And don't
be hard on yourself when you aren't feeling
it. There will be better days and better times.
Prioritize yourself.

Getting Creative with Your Setup

Props and toys are your pals. With the right set-up,
I'm of the mind that masturbation can work for
any body. Thinking ahead to what you may need
in a space to make yourself feel good is critical!
Especially for folks who may need assistance from
others to prepare themselves/their space for solo
time. Setting your space up for sexy time means
you have nothing to stress over when you're
getting down to business. It also helps you get into
a headspace that feels sexual. Feeling secure and
sexy in your environment, surrounded by any and
all of the things you may need, just makes space
for you to relax and give into whatever feels good.
Light some candles, friend, you deserve it.

sex toys explained

BUILD YOUR TOYKIT

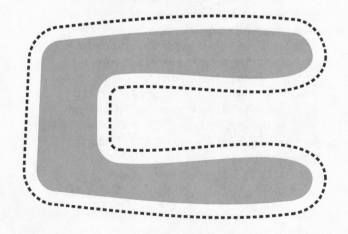

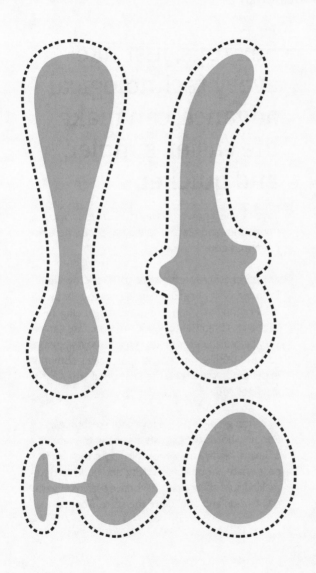

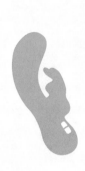

Sex toys, just like every technological advance, can make life easier, simpler, and quicker.

Toys can be a powerful way to push your own boundaries and reach a speed or space where no finger has gone before.

For purchasing your first (or 50th) sex toy, we've included a list of recommended sex toy shops. While shops may appear intimidating, being able to see and hold the toys prior to purchase can be very helpful in determining what is most appealing to you. Just like with dating apps, seeing something in person is a smart way to suss out if you want it inside of you.

Sex shop employees are invaluable resources. People who work at sex shops are, in the majority of cases, highly knowledgeable about their work, passionate about sex positivity, and dedicated to making sure their customers have a great experience inside and outside of the store. They're not

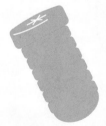

there to judge you or laugh at you. They will be able to help you most effectively if you communicate clearly what you're looking for, or the fact that you have no idea what you're looking for.

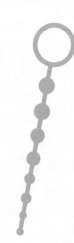

If you are ever in a sex shop where you feel as though you are being judged for your sexual orientation or preferences, leave immediately. While you may feel anxious or embarrassed about buying a sex toy, no one else should make you feel that way. When in doubt, sex toys can be purchased everywhere from online sex shops, such as the ones we recommend below.

Rules of Play

Always clean your toys after each use with soap and water. Toy wipes are fantastic for the discreet or the lazy. You can even use condoms or latex gloves over your toys.

If you're lubing up (always a great choice), make sure to use water-based lubes for any silicone- or rubber-based toys. When in doubt, use water-based.

Pro-tip: Park your charger near your bed. You're going to need it.

Your sex toy will be more intimate with your body than most things or people. So finding the right one is pretty darn important.

Before even reading through the shop options below, we suggest that you do some soul-searching about what experience you're looking for. Do you want to ask questions or personal opinions? Do you have a specific brand or toy in mind? Are you the type of person who likes to see every possible option before choosing one? Are you looking for a specific aesthetic? What's your price range?

Amazon.com is understandably the internet's favorite online sex toy shop. Delivery is fast and dependable. But buyers beware, it's really hard to verify the quality of the sex toys and how they have been stored! Also, we don't love supporting The Man (and his unethical practices) with our personal sexplorations. Here, we've collected some of our favorite shops that both walk the walk and talk the talk of loving your body.

The Classics

These are the Golden Girls of the sex toy world, the timeless beauts that have earned their mentions in pop culture, that have been around the block before feminism was fashionable, and were trailblazers for sex-positive culture. They carry a wide, wide range of toys and brands, and have full online shops no matter where you are.

The Pleasure Chest
$$–$$$

If you're a *Sex and the City* watcher, then you've heard of the Pleasure Chest. If Charlotte trusted the Pleasure Chest with her orgasms, you probably can too.

Good Vibrations and Babeland
$$–$$$

Good Vibrations was founded to provide a safe, welcoming alternative to traditional adult stores. Since then, it has expanded to include toys for all gender expressions. Babeland is its little sibling, branded and geared towards a younger population.

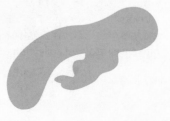

The Locals

We're a bit biased toward your local mom-and-pop sex-toy shop. Local sex toy shops are reliably chock-full of passionate, educated individuals, as well as well-curated collections. These shops are amazing choices for sex-toy newbies looking for some guidance, or sex-toy masters looking to expand their collection. Often friendly and welcoming, each shop has their own voice or aesthetic. They often have monthly sex-education workshops as well, and can be a wonderful way to support or connect with your neighborhood sex-positive community.

Depending on where you live, you'll likely have to find your own neighborhood version. We recommend a quick Google search with key words like "sex-positive" and a look at the reviews and pictures. But here are a few to get you started, and they all have online shops!

Early to Bed
$$
Andersonville, Chicago and online
Vibe: Kitschy and artsy. Lots of fun personality, but also lots of knowledge! Passionately sex-positive and lots of LGBTQIA+ pride. Great for all genders, with a well-stocked collection of gender gear.

Sugar
$$

Hampden, Baltimore and online
Vibe: Well-organized, well-lit, and very educational.
It doesn't have a strong personality, but sometimes
that is exactly what you want out of a sex-toy shop.

Shag... A Sexy Shop
$$$

Brooklyn, New York and online
Vibe: Curated and femme, it leans towards a
lifestyle brand with lingerie from local designers,
candles, and jewelry.

She Bop
$$$

Clinton, Portland; Boise, Portland; and online
Vibe: Well-organized, educational, and established,
but also fun and quirky. Originally started as a
sex-positive shop for women, it has now expanded
to support all bodies and gender expressions.

Come as You Are
$–$$$

Toronto, Online-Only
Vibe: The world's only worker-owned
co-operative sex toy shop. Extremely queer-in-
clusive. Anti-capitalist and sex-positive, with an
amazing return policy.

Your options include...

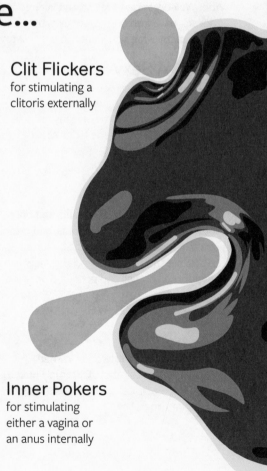

Clit Flickers
for stimulating a
clitoris externally

Inner Pokers
for stimulating
either a vagina or
an anus internally

Butt Pluggers
for stimulating the
anus internally through
gentle dilation

Strokers
for external stimulation
of either a penis or an
enlarged clitoris

Prostate Prodders
angled for prostate
stimulation through
the anus

Clit Flickers

stimulate externally on or around the clitoris. Size and shape can be anything from a small toy that travels well (like a simple bullet or the Fin by Dame Products) to much larger and more powerful toys (think Hitachi wand). Toys can have multiple speeds, patterns, or rhythms of vibration. Generally used for external stimulation for the clitoris, they are easily combined with penetrators, sleeves, or butt plugs. Factors to consider include intensity of vibrations, different patterns or rhythms, and level of sound that the toy makes. Vibrators tend to be silicone-based.

Inner Pokers

stimulate a vagina or an anus internally. Dildos, like penises, come in many different shapes and sizes. Unlike penises, some vibrate! Here, it's all about finding what suits you, but make sure that if you have anal plans, your toy has a flared base. For those of you with a clitoris considering a multi-tasker like a rabbit vibrator: many find that having two separate toys, one for vaginal penetration and one for clitoral stimulation, tends to fit their bodies more readily than finding the perfect 2-in-1 shampoo and conditioner.

Strokers

envelop a penis or an elongated clitoris as
they are moved up and down the shaft. The
inside material is often textured with raised patterns
for stimulation. Factors to consider when selecting
a sleeve include the type of entrance, length and
width, and material. The inside material ranges
from jelly (very affordable, but may come with a
particular texture and smell) to silicone, to rubber.
Some vibrate. While a close-ended toy can provide
more suction and a tighter feel, cleaning these toys
can be more difficult than cleaning open-ended
toys. Strokers can be wonderful for transmasculine
masturbation—just find one that fits, like the Sexy
Pills Blue Valentine or the Shotpocket Sleeve.

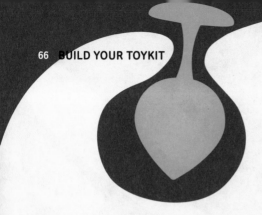

Butt Pluggers

can be inserted and left in, hands-free, during masturbation to increase pressure and pleasure. Their characteristic flared base keeps the plug from traveling up the rectum, and the tapered end makes for easy insertion. A handle can also be used to manipulate the plug for extra feels. Some plugs even vibrate! Length ranges from around 2 to 3 inches, to up to 6 inches. With regards to the material, consider the length and type of use. Plugs that are worn for longer should be made of the more flexible silicone, while glass and body-safe metals can be heated or cooled for temperature play. Cleaning is very important for plugs, to deal with bacterial growth and small traces of poop.

Prostate Prodders

stimulate the prostate gland through the anus. Because the prostate is located approximately 3 to 4 inches past the beginning of the anal canal, it's a hard place to reach with fingers alone. The right toy can do wonders, although it may take some trial and error to find the perfect length, size, and shape. Hands-on massagers can be used to more powerfully stimulate the prostate through motion and positioning. Hands-free models will stay put, leaving your hands free to focus on other things. Don't forget to lubricate thyself!

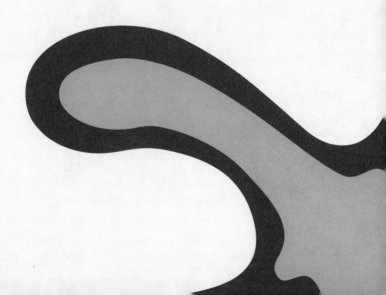

checking in with yourself

post-coital tristesse

THE SADs

You know that feeling when you finish a really good book or movie and you get sad?

The same thing might happen after masturbation, and it's called post-coital tristesse (PCT). People are not too sure why it happens, but many are affected by it. Some describe it as a slight feeling of despair after orgasm.

Here you are, fingers or toy covered in your own fluids, unclothed, after the fervor of a climax. It's like those romantic movies that end on that insanely happy note when against all odds the star-crossed lovers are united... and the credits roll and you're back in your parents' basement alone on a Saturday night and have half a mind to weep all over the afghan. You go from all the happy feels to hello mundanity. What a mood killer.

PCT is a phenomenon well-documented all the way back to Ancient Rome, and people have known about it since people have been masturbating and having sex. All these years later, there still isn't very much knowledge of why it happens. The most commonly accepted theory is pretty similar to the movie analogy: what goes up must come down.

In an ideal world, every time one of us came on our own, a ceiling of gold balloons and confetti would fall and Oprah would explode out of the ground and point to you majestically and say,

"GOOD FOR YOU! Taking charge of your pleasure, exploring your body. Good on you!"

It would only be fair to counter all of society's intrusive toxicity inherited from convoluted nonsense.

But Oprah's busy, so the job falls to you. If you're feeling some PCT after orgasm, give yourself a good, long hug (I suggest with a body pillow), you wonderful special duck.

Remind yourself that you are natural. Your body is just as it's supposed to be. You are just as you are meant to be. This PCT thing will pass very quickly, while all the benefits of your lovin' will last.

GUILT

it happens

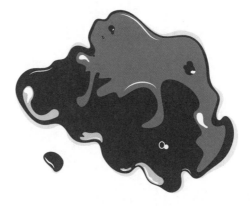

The thing about masturbation is you have to make the first move. The first time I masturbated, I was lying on my back, head propped up with pillows. I reached for the cold metal of my newly-purchased vibrator. I pressed a button, felt the sharp buzz against my fingers, and... tossed it off the bed.

Somewhere along the road of insecurity, I had convinced myself that my body was too much of some things—too large, too inexperienced—and too little of other things—not attractive enough, not experienced enough—to deserve pleasure. I felt ashamed of my body—how could I deserve something that made this body feel good?

For people like me, guilt keeps us from masturbating.

We teeter on the edge, trying to convince ourselves to take the risk, but the shame and guilt we feel rises, keeping us from the act of letting go that makes masturbation a pleasurable and profound act.

Even for those who have crossed the barrier, armed with their own vibrators, lube, and courage, guilt can be the product of masturbation. Thanks to centuries of religious and cultural norms, masturbation is seen as a major transgression, a solo act revealed as a crime against yourself and your community.

A number of significant religions condemn masturbation as "unnatural" due to its lack of reproductive capacity, and paint masturbation as a dirty, perverted, or selfish act. With religion serving as a moral and behavioral guide for many families and communities, guilt is woven into acts of self pleasure from the very beginning.

Many people are drawn to masturbate at a young age, instinct and sensation guiding a natural exploration of the body and its marvelous capacity (see page 92). In a society that tries to child-proof access to information about sex, many people's early experiences with masturbation leave them uncertain and seeking guidance about what the new sensations mean.

What happens when a child goes to their parents, guardians, or trusted adults seeking answers about masturbation, and the adult's primary thought is children shouldn't masturbate? In many cases, parents will react with concern, disgust, or condemnation. Sometimes, when children grow up, it's hard for them to masturbate, even as adults, without perceiving the act as somehow dirty or wrong.

Guilt is also sometimes related to masturbation within relationships.

Even for people who feel comfortable with masturbation as a solo practice, conventional beliefs around monogamous romantic relationships dictate that one's sexual desires and needs should be completely satisfied by one's partner. Masturbation can feel like an accusation against your partner or lover - why can't I give you what your body needs? Why am I not enough for you?

The desire to masturbate while in an exclusive sexual or romantic relationship can provoke the fear that either you or your partner is inadequate — if my partner is supposed to fulfill all of my sexual needs, why do I still want to masturbate? If my partner finds out I want to masturbate, will they think that I don't want to have sex with them, or that the sex we have isn't enough for me?

Many people attempt to protect their partners or themselves from feelings of inadequacy by hiding the fact that they masturbate. By hiding masturbation, we withhold precious information from our partners about what makes us feel good.

When it comes to guilt surrounding masturbation in a relationship, talking to your partner is key to resolution. An open conversation about masturbation not only fosters honesty and open communication in your relationship, but can also allow you to more fully explore your sexual experiences together.

One of the most insidious qualities of guilt is how isolating the feeling can be.

Take the isolation of guilt and add the intimacy and often solo nature of masturbation, and you end up with a situation that can occur without any external feedback or checkpoints. The simplest way to address masturbation-related guilt, while challenging and terrifying, is to share your experience with someone else.

If you give yourself permission to share this guilt with someone you trust, you open yourself up to understanding that others share this experience, and allow yourself to receive affirmation that a desire to masturbate is not only normal, but completely healthy and positive. This reality check of learning that you are not alone is key to moving past guilt.

An external perspective, personal or professional, can be extremely useful for identifying where your guilt is coming from.

While a friend or a partner may be able to provide positive feedback and support in these situations, it can feel intimidating to open this conversation with someone close to you. You might feel scared that they will judge you for masturbating or for your feelings of guilt. In this case, consider reaching out to a physician or a mental health practitioner.

A professional within these fields will be able to reassure you that your sexuality and experience with masturbation are coming from a natural, healthy place. They may also have useful advice or methods for helping shift your perspective on masturbation.

If you do not currently have access to a medical professional, there are several sex-education and sex-positive organizations that operate across the U.S., including Planned Parenthood, the Sexuality Information and Education Council of the United States, and the American Sexual Health Association. These organizations have tons of information available on healthy masturbation. Several of them also provide hotlines for asking questions about sex and sexual health.

Having someone else try to ease your feelings of guilt can only go so far.

Ultimately, what may need to change is the conversation you have with yourself about masturbation. It took me many more nights of lying in that bed, vibrator on the floor, and many difficult and vulnerable conversations with people I loved, before I could give myself permission to start masturbating, free of guilt and self-judgment.

Feeling guilty about masturbating reaffirms a false narrative that your body's natural instincts are wrong, and that the desire to masturbate means that there is something wrong with you. If you can shift this narrative to one where masturbation is considered natural and normal, guilt can move out of the way of your exploration and pleasure.

hitting the books

the history of a stigma

DESTR

OF CIVILIZ

2,600-year-old depiction
of a Satyr masturbating

Attributed to Kleophrades Painter
500–480 BCE, Terracotta

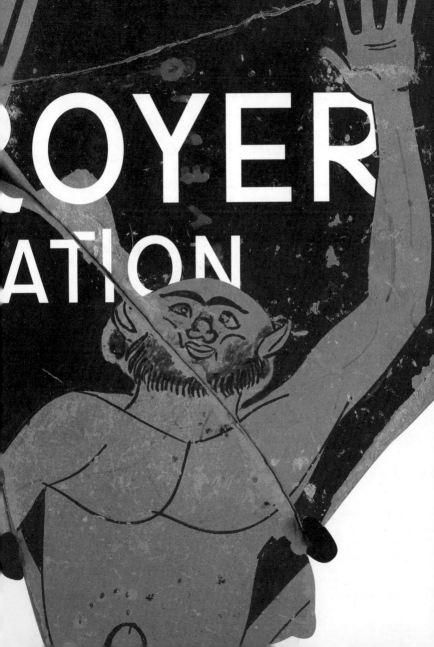

Alex, my partner, thought he invented masturbation at age 13.

And there you have it, the reason that masturbation has been part of the human story since the very beginning.

Across culture and time, independently or with help, humans have found their way to their genitalia. In the Ancient Egyptian Heliopolis creation myth, dating to between 2,780–2,250 BCE, Atum, the first god, created all other gods through masturbation. Seven bronze dildos dating from 200 BCE were found in a Han dynasty tomb in China. Through the 15th and 16th centuries, aristocrats in both China and Europe possessed ornate dildos, some made of lacquered wood and some cast in precious metals. The Ancient Greek physician Hippocrates and the Ancient Roman physician Galen believed masturbation was essential to remove unused "seed" in order to avoid blockages in the human bodily system. Galen, the dominant medical authority of the Romans, proposed masturbation as a remedy for insanity in women.

Galen argued that sexual release was as necessary as urination or bowel movements.

Given this long history, where did the stigma against masturbation come from? Why do we feel ashamed or guilty about touching ourselves when our ancestors did so for all of human history? It turns out that the story of the self-stimulation stigma is also a story of the birth of society, with all of its insecurities and anxieties.

The birth of the stigma against masturbation paralleled a growing fear about the finiteness of humans. If semen was finite, each act of masturbation was an individual's contribution to starving society. Masturbation cast semen on useless bedsheets instead of within waiting wombs. As far as society was concerned, more masturbation meant fewer babies. (To be fair they also believed in the idea of the homunculus, where sperm consisted of literal mini-humans. Some went as far as to argue that masturbation was murder). Therefore, every time someone wanked off, they were threatening society's survival.

IMAGE: Ancient Egyptian papyrus of Atum, the first god, masturbating the other gods into existence.[1]

c. 29,000 BC, oldest stone phallus
likely used as a dildo.

Religions showcased the earliest prohibition of
masturbation as a social defense mechanism. In 500
BCE, the Christian Church prohibited masturbation
because it wasted sperm that could be used for
procreation. Judaism also held similar reasonings
for prohibiting male masturbation. It demonstrated
admirable logical coherence, though, by allowing
female masturbation because it didn't waste semen.
However, it wasn't until the late 1700s that the
stigma infiltrated public culture.

The widespread stigma against masturbation we
see in America today has surprisingly secular origins
in the Enlightenment. The secular stigma against
masturbation appeared during the rapid urbaniza-
tion of the Enlightenment in the late 1700s. For the
first time, Europe lived in packed cities, and it was
afraid for its own survival. Urban society was born,
and it fervently encouraged the ideal of the rational
man as a guide for behavior, as one would in such
close quarters.

Masturbation simply did not fit the new image of an ideal man (or neighbor) in complete control of his desires and urges.[2]

Masturbation became associated with physical debilitation, illness, and insanity. Samuel-August Tissot's 1760 *Onanism* proclaimed that losing 1 ounce of semen was equivalent to losing 40 ounces of blood. It described a whole host of ailments born of this depraved practice, including hysterical fit and violent cramps in the neck and back. In 1812, Benjamin Rush linked masturbation to insanity, seminal weakness, impotence, pulmonary consumption, dimness of sight, vertigo, epilepsy, loss of memory, and death.[2] In 1828, Joseph Henri Reveille-Parise called it "the destroyer of civilization," as masturbators were charged with enfeebling the young men and future fathers, and the manpower of king and country.

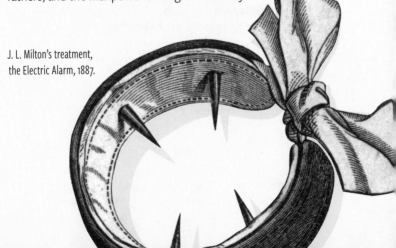

J. L. Milton's treatment, the Electric Alarm, 1887.

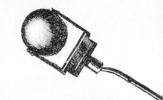

It was as if you could destroy a nation by handing out enough free smut.

Parallel to these new "scientific" discoveries, Victorian cities invented the concept of good manners. Its citizens, the newly created bourgeoisie, prided themselves on their unique morality. They were not idle like the elites nor animalistic like the masses. They were restrained, and defined themselves by "the control of impulses."[3] Modesty was born and people began bathing clothed for the first time. And if nudity was forbidden, then jacking one's bean(stalk) was also frowned upon. The new society was restrained. It was proud to say it did not enjoy sex, but bore the burden patriotically. And it went to great lengths to protect its children from the dangers of touching oneself (see The Electric Alarm on page 89).

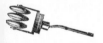

Perhaps because of the birth of psychoanalysis, or perhaps due to the bourgeoisie's newfound stability, the 1880s finally witnessed the beginning of a decline in the masturbation slander. The tide was turning.

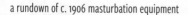

a rundown of c. 1906 masturbation equipment

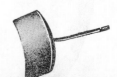

It began with the backpedaling by many strong opponents of masturbation, who retracted arguments that masturbation was dangerous but settled for an "it's still gross." During this time, it became common for unmarried women to be treated for hysteria with genital massages by their doctor, a quasi-return to Ancient Greece. One theory holds that the first vibrators were created in 1880 for doctors to treat women for hysteria. Vibrators would later become commercially available in the early 1900s.

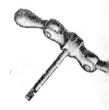

Masturbation was beginning to reclaim its role as a component of health.

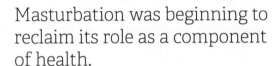

The rise of sexual liberation continued, powered by the shocking revelation that most people already masturbated. Katherine Davis's 1929 survey of 2,200 women revealed that over 65% of unmarried women and 40% of married women masturbated, while two-thirds of them were embarrassed by that fact.

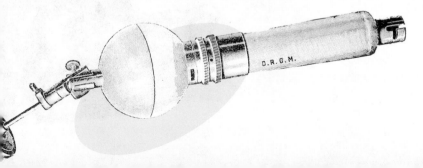

Alfred Kinsey's 1950s survey showed that 92% of men and 62% of women masturbated.

In the 1960s, the vibrator became increasingly popular within households. The Masters and Johnson research team advocated masturbation to help marital relationships and general health, especially for women during menstruation.

It is possible that the new commercial availability of female contraception, such as the pill in the 1960s and the legalization of abortion in the 1970s, contributed to the masturbation liberation. Cis women could be sexual beings without sacrificing their way of life. And that meant taking sex into their own hands openly.

Sprinkles Banana Split
PJ Linden, 2010

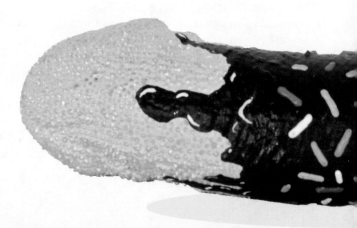

And finally, here we are today.

For the most part, America is much more supportive of a healthy solo sex life than it has ever been. We can order the delivery of our next favorite diddler with a click of a button. It's easier to watch free porn than to watch a free movie. But it's also a whole mess of opinions, with people still shaming each other and themselves for participating in an ancient human tradition. But then again, it's always been a mess of opinions. Because back when half of England was locking up vulvas in chastity belts and tying bells and whistles and needles to penises to avoid unconscious erections, there were also those dirty deviants who were depraved enough to pick the locks.

This one's for them.

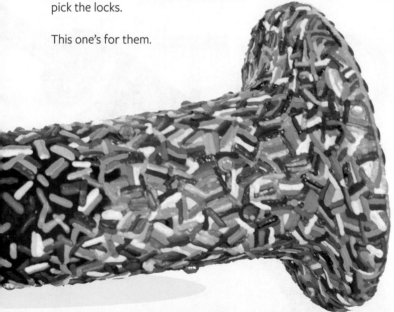

childhood masturbation is very normal!

DON'T FREAK OUT

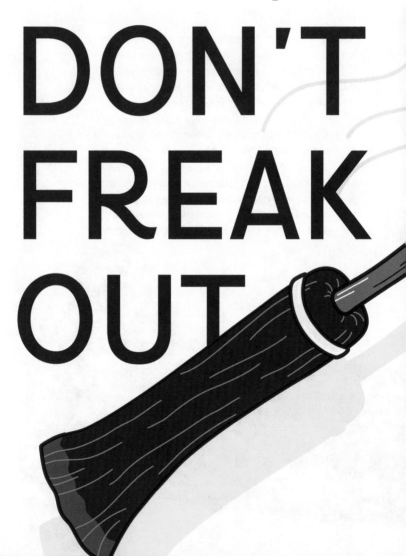

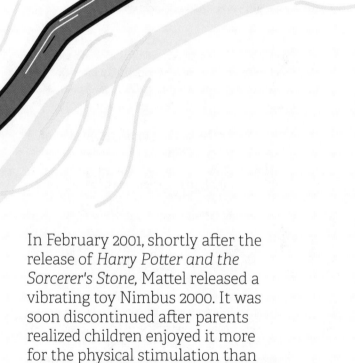

In February 2001, shortly after the release of *Harry Potter and the Sorcerer's Stone,* Mattel released a vibrating toy Nimbus 2000. It was soon discontinued after parents realized children enjoyed it more for the physical stimulation than for the Quidditch.

Children begin masturbating between the ages of 2 and 6.

Not just some children, most children.

We know that sounds pretty surprising, but remember that children are operating in a world completely different from ours. It's a pretty insane thing to be born into this world, to go from not existing in one moment to very much existing.

Right around the ages of 2 through 6, children are beginning to learn the boundaries between what is their own body and what is the larger world. Which logically would lead to exploration of all the weird nooks and crannies of their newfound own-ness of their bodies, including their private parts.

It's necessary to remember that their world is completely devoid of the social context and conno- tations we are so deeply immersed in and aware of. For them, masturbation isn't about sex. It isn't sexual at all; in fact, it's more sensual. Sensational. It is a pure exploration of the relationship between their physical bodies and their emotional experi- ences, another way of learning about themselves.

The other crucial component of this self-exploration is how the adults around the child react. Reacting with shock or embarrassment can teach children to be ashamed or embarrassed of contact with their genitals, which can negatively impact their relationship with their body in the future.

So how could you react if you happen on a child masturbating?

Focus on the context rather than the act. Explain to the child that masturbation, like going to the bathroom, is to be done in private. You can also try to distract or redirect the child's attention.

When should you call the pediatrician?

When it is so frequent that it interferes with daily life. It is completely normal for children to masturbate a few times daily, weekly, or monthly; however if you feel that their behavior is impeding their daily activities, it never hurts to call the pediatrician. Another sign that you should consult a doctor is if the child is unable to be distracted, or if the child is using objects that might be harmful.

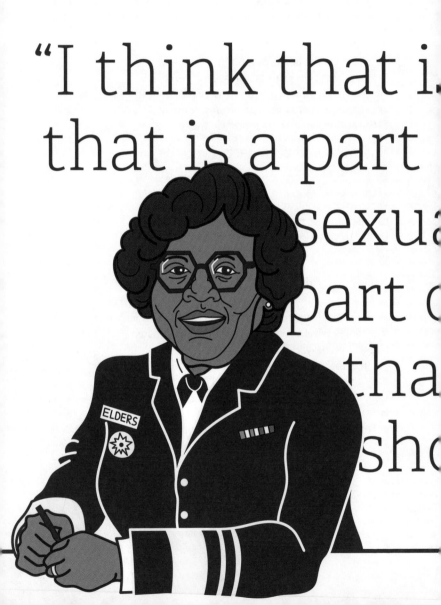

"I think that i.
that is a part

sexua

part o

tha

sho

something
f human
ity and it's a
f something
perhaps
ld be taught."

Joycelyn Elders, the first African-American and the
second woman U.S. Surgeon General, was fired by
Bill Clinton (ironically) over her suggestion that
masturbation should be addressed in schools.

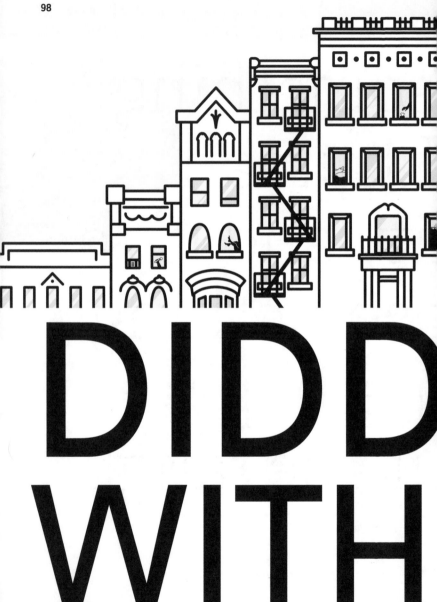

DIDD
WITH

In 2009, Dr. Debby Herbernick and her colleagues gathered data from 5,865 people from across the United States about their masturbation habits.

When it comes to a topic full of hearsay, word-of-mouth, myths, and superstitions, data is a gift to humanity. Within these numbers, lines, and graphs is a peek into the bedrooms of Americans across all ages.

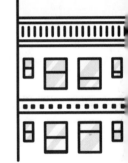

LING DATA

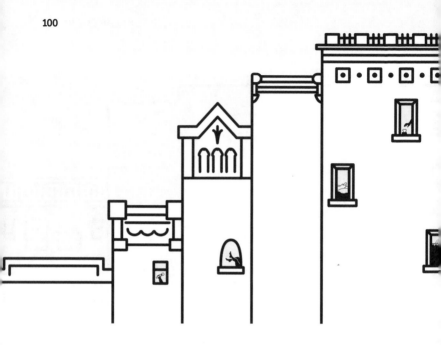

A few things to keep in mind as you delve into the following graphs:

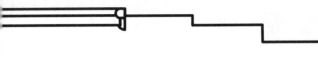

1   The data is collected from over 5,865 individuals ranging from ages 14 to 94. It is not the rate of masturbation of the same group of individuals as they age. The increase or decrease in monthly masturbation across these groups is affected not only by their biological age, but also their cultural perspective and upbringing.

2   A multitude of factors affect how often someone masturbates or whether they masturbate at all. Rate of masturbation does not directly translate to sexual appetite.

3   These numbers reflect what was reported by people voluntarily. It is likely that the true proportion of people who masturbate is higher, as masturbation is one of the most underreported sexual acts.

4   The survey does not dig into sexual orientation, nor gender beyond (presumably cisgender) "men" and "women".

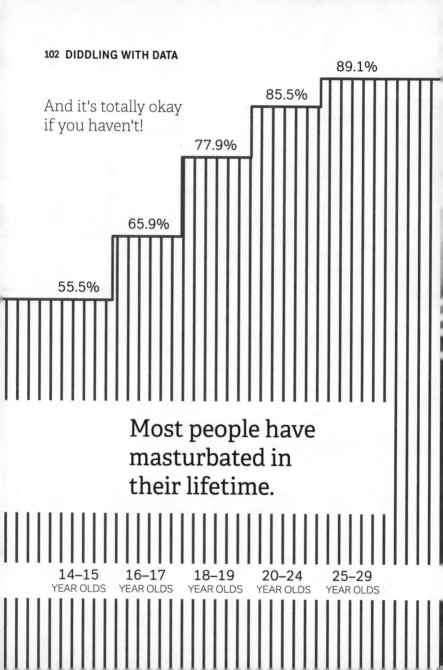

And it's totally okay
if you haven't!

89.1%

85.5%

77.9%

65.9%

55.5%

Most people have
masturbated in
their lifetime.

14–15
YEAR OLDS

16–17
YEAR OLDS

18–19
YEAR OLDS

20–24
YEAR OLDS

25–29
YEAR OLDS

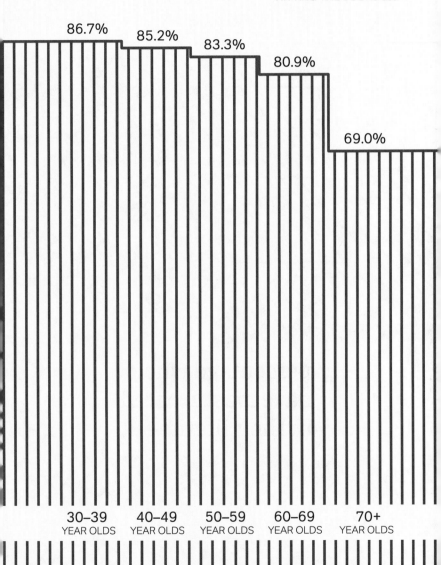

86.7%   85.2%   83.3%   80.9%

69.0%

30–39   40–49   50–59   60–69   70+
YEAR OLDS   YEAR OLDS   YEAR OLDS   YEAR OLDS   YEAR OLDS

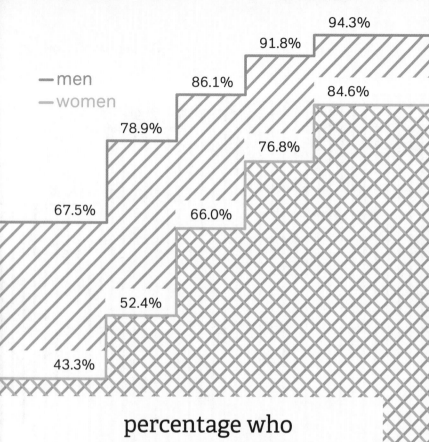

percentage who
have masturbated
in their lifetime

—men
—women

94.3%

91.8%

86.1%

84.6%

78.9%

76.8%

67.5%

66.0%

52.4%

43.3%

14–15
YEAR OLDS

16–17
YEAR OLDS

18–19
YEAR OLDS

20–24
YEAR OLDS

25–29
YEAR OLDS

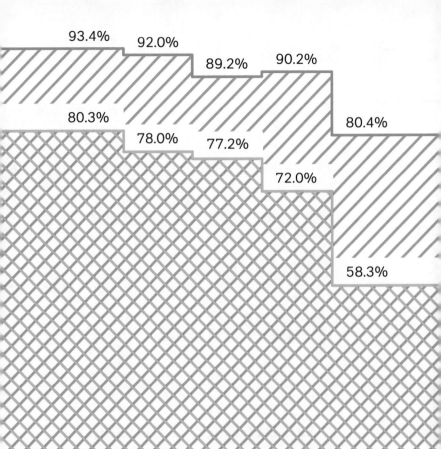

| 30–39 | 40–49 | 50–59 | 60–69 | 70+ |
| YEAR OLDS | YEAR OLDS | YEAR OLDS | YEAR OLDS | YEAR OLDS |

93.4%
92.0%
89.2%
90.2%
80.3%
78.0%
77.2%
72.0%
80.4%
58.3%

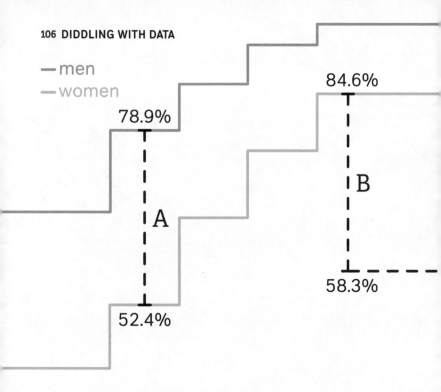

—men
—women

78.9%

84.6%

B

A

52.4%

58.3%

On average, more men
have masturbated than
women in their lifetime.

16–17
YEAR OLDS

25–29
YEAR OLDS

Because these numbers reflect the percentage of survey respondents who have ever masturbated throughout their entire life, they also reflect the influence of the time on people's behaviors. In other words, the amount a 70 year-old has ever masturbated in their lifetime can reflect the attitudes of the time. The data indicate:

A At the average age at which people had sex for the first time in 2009, way more men had masturbated than women. This discrepancy could greatly affect the dynamics of the sexual encounters between men and women during this age range. It implies an unequal level of comfort with one's body between the two partners.

B There is a huge rise in the number of women that have masturbated in their lifetime from the age brackets 70+ to the age bracket of 25–29 years. This rise might be connected with an increasing social acceptance of feminine sexuality.

70+
YEAR OLDS

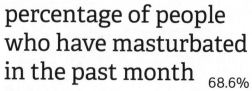

— men
— women

percentage of people who have masturbated in the past month

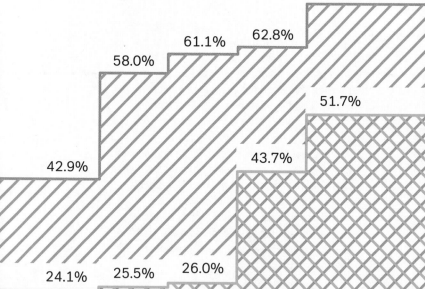

68.6%

62.8%

61.1%

58.0%

51.7%

43.7%

42.9%

26.0%

25.5%

24.1%

| 14–15 YEAR OLDS | 16–17 YEAR OLDS | 18–19 YEAR OLDS | 20–24 YEAR OLDS | 25–29 YEAR OLDS |

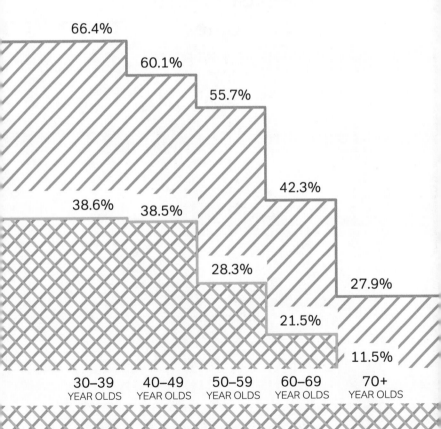

66.4%
60.1%
55.7%
42.3%
38.6%
38.5%
28.3%
27.9%
21.5%
11.5%

30–39
YEAR OLDS

40–49
YEAR OLDS

50–59
YEAR OLDS

60–69
YEAR OLDS

70+
YEAR OLDS

—men
—women

More men reported masturbating in the past month than women.

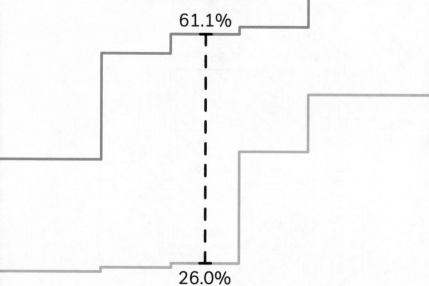

61.1%

26.0%

18–19
YEAR OLDS

Overall, the data indicate that people between the ages of 25 and 29 masturbate the most frequently, with a gradual decline as people age. The data also indicate that women masturbate far less frequently than men in the age range of 18 to 19 years old.

Crucially, this age range is when most people are beginning their adult lives, whether in college or the workforce, and often entails an increase in sexual experiences. Like the previous case, in this age range, the huge difference in masturbation frequency between men and women may signal a difference in bodily comfort levels, and may affect the dynamic of het sexual experiences.

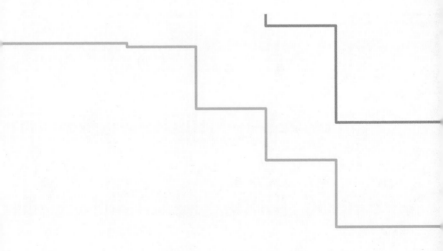

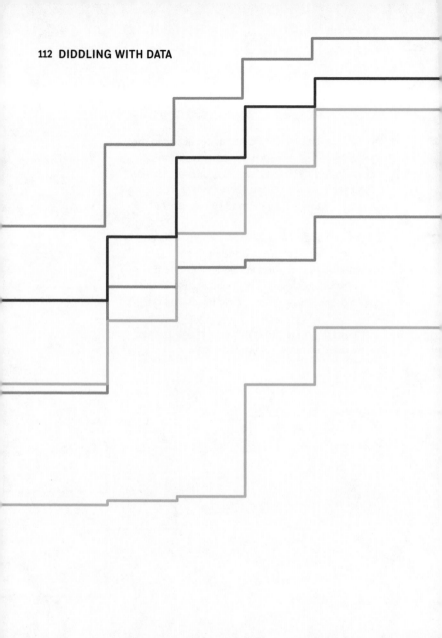

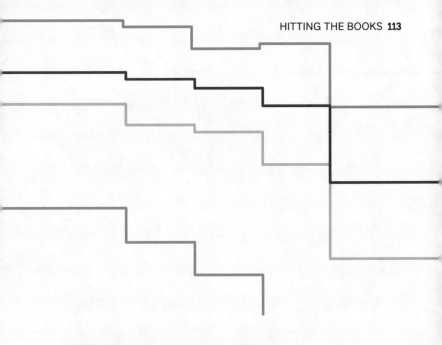

We know, we know. We nerded out a bit with the data here.

But here's the deal: you've got the cold, hard numbers now. Consider yourself armed against all the hearsay and mumblings of the world. If you don't remember anything else from these pages, remember this: most people masturbate.

And that's a fact.

finishing you off

THANKS FOR COMING

At the end of the day, I can't figure out if sex is the most important thing in the world or the least important thing in the world.

The hard truth at the heart of this book is that we aren't trained to accept ourselves as we are. It's really hard to do. And the moments that count aren't the easy or loud ones, but the quiet moments by yourself, when you might find yourself feeling some sort of negativity towards your specific mash-up of pieces, what makes you tick, and how your body works. The quiet moments when you question the way you are, or wish you were different.

Sure, masturbation is about all the fun physical and emotional feels your body can give you, but it's also about being alone with parts of yourself, mental and physical, that no one else can make you love. The normal parts and the strange parts. The parts you haven't talked about with anyone else. And the parts you have only just begun to figure out yourself.

It takes real hard work to learn to accept yourself. And it's never going to be perfect. But it's going to get a lot easier. We promise.

So remember:

1. Most people masturbate.
2. Touch yourself if you want to.
3. And don't let anyone mess with the wonderful weirdo you are. Including yourself.

ACKNO WLEDG MENTS

Bang was anything but a solo act.

To Nina Chausow, Alex Tait, Clare Edgeman, Leah Holmes, Sam Dusing, Patrick Wiedeman, Rebecca Bedell, Lafayette Matthews, Andrew Gurza, and Angus Andrews: thank you for being vulnerable, brave, and open. Thank you for digging deep and letting everyone into some of your most private experiences. This book is built out of your honesty.

To Francis Van Ganson, Jennifer Shyue, Megan Pryce, and Daphne Weinstein: thank you for your generosity with your design eyes, literary brains, and grammar superpowers when I couldn't even see straight anymore. This book would be in far worse shape without you.

To independent bookstores and sex toy shops including Uncharted Books, Quimby's Bookstore NYC, Atomic Books, Spoonbill and Sugartown Books, Shag...a sexy shop, and Early to Bed, thank you for believing in this book back when it was a 'lil ol' zine. It wouldn't have become a book without your zine shelves, your study spaces, and your radical support of weirdos like me.

To the sex-positive writers and researches before me, and the sex educators at high schools and colleges, thanks for fighting the good fight.

To my parents, Hong Liu and Zhimin Wang, for being open-minded and holding space for different ways of being a citizen of the world. To Jenny, for always keeping the gray couch open.

To Alex, for believing in me, always. I wouldn't be shitting half as many rainbows without you.

And lastly, to Peppercorn, who constantly demonstrates that genitals aren't a big deal by licking her butthole on my desk.

By the way, a portion of the proceeds will be donated to Advocates for Youth, an amazing national nonprofit that works alongside youth leaders and their adult allies to fight for sexual health, rights and justice.

SOURCES

falsehoods

The Secret Companion, R J Brodie London, 1845. Credit: Wellcome Collection. Attribution 4.0 International (CC BY 4.0)

Miller, Kelsey. "15 Masturbation Myths We Somehow Still Believe." Refinery29, Refinery29, Mar. 20, 2016.

1 Herbenick D, Reece M, Schick V, Sanders SA, Dodge B, Fortenberry JD. Sexual behaviors, relationships, and perceived health status among adult women in the United States: results from a national probability sample. J Sex Med. 2010; 7 Suppl 5:277 290.

perks of playing

Masturbation, plannedparenthood.org

master debate class

Saturn Apollo Program, Marshall Space Flight Center, 1961.

guilt

Aneja J, Grover S, Avasthi A, Mahajan S, Pokhrel P, Triveni D. Can masturbatory guilt lead to severe psychopathology: a case series. Indian J Psychol Med. 2015;37(1):81–86.

Hungrige, Angela. "Women's Masturbation: an Exploration of the Influence of Shame, Guilt, and Religiosity." Texas Woman's University, Texas Woman's University, 2016.

Katehakis, Alexandra. "Childhood Trauma and Masturbation." *Psychology Today*, 6 Feb. 2015.

Ley, David J. "Overcoming Religious Sexual Shame." Psychology Today, 23 Aug. 2017.

MacGinley, M, Breckenridge, J, Mowll, J. A scoping review of adult survivors' experiences of shame following sexual abuse in childhood. Health Soc Care Community. 2019; 27: 1135– 1146.

Prendergast, William E. The Merry-Go-Round of Sexual Abuse: Identifying and Treating Survivors. Haworth Press, 1993.

Ramos, Marciana Julia. *Masturbation and Relationship Satisfaction*, thesis, May 2013; Denton, Texas. University of North Texas Libraries, UNT Digital Library,

Werder, Corinne. "Sex After Trauma: How Masturbation Can Help You Heal." GO Magazine, 12 Oct. 2018.

destroyer of civilization

500–480 BCE, Terracotta. Attributed to Kleophrades Painter. The J. Paul Getty Museum, Villa Collection, Malibu, California

[1] Mels van Driel. With the Hand: a Cultural History of Masturbation. Reaktion, 2012.

[2] Julie Peakman,"From Onanism to Spending." The Pleasure's All Mine: a History of Perverse Sex, Reaktion Books, 2016, pp. 45–73.

Hohle Fels phallus, Prehistory Museum, Blaubeuren.

Illustration showing various instruments used in vibratory massage. Round or square Concussor Plates, Concussor Rollers, Balls and Discs, Roller with rotating cylinders and ebonite, Rotating hammers and Centrifugal Vibrator. Credit: Wellcome Collection. Attribution 4.0 International (CC BY 4.0)

diddling with data

"Sexual Behavior in the United States: Results from a National Probability Sample of Men and Women Ages 14–94" Herbenick, Debby et al. The Journal of Sexual Medicine, Volume 7, 255 - 265

don't freak out

Klass, Perri. "Why Is Children's Masturbation Such a Secret?" The New York Times, Dec. 10, 2018.

"Masturbation." HealthyChildren.org, American Academy of Pediatrics, Nov. 2009.

COLOPHON

We try to support people of under-represented backgrounds when we can, and that includes type designers.

The cover is set in Lelo, designed by Katharina Köhler. Our titles are set in Ferpal, a typeface designed by Silvia Fernández Palomar. Our subheadlines are set in Tondo, a typeface designed by Veronika Burian. Our pull quotes are set in Adelle, a typeface designed by Veronika Burian and José Scaglione. Our body text is set in Freight Sans, designed by Joshua Darden. The subheadlines of Falsehoods are set in Amador is designed by Jim Parkinson.

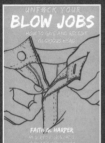
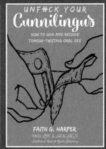
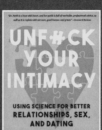
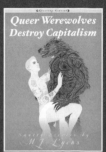

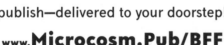
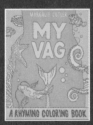
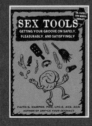
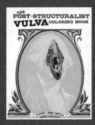
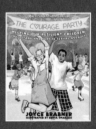